Mastering Your Sugar levels

by

Eugene I.Warren

Table Of Content

INTRODUCTION

CHAPTER 1

- Blood Sugar Relevance to the Body
- Why did my blood sugar Spike?

CHAPTER 2

- Glucagon
- Analysis of Achieving Insulin Sensitivity

- How eating food in the right order will help you lose weight
- Strategies of mindful eating and portion control

CHAPTER 3

- For Stable Blood Glucose: Diet and Nutrition
- Nutrition for Blood Glucose Stability

- Meal planning and some sample menus

- Glycemic Index (GI):

CHAPTER 4

- Microbiome

- What is a macronutrient?

- Should a diabetic avoid fats?

- Fiber's Essential Function in Blood Glucose Management

CHAPTER 5

- Sleep Quality and its Impact on Blood Glucose Levels
- Stress Management and Blood Glucose Harmony
- Nurturing healthy weight management
- Blood Sugar Symptoms
- How can I be tested for diabetes?

CHAPTER 6

- Understanding signs and symptoms
- Managing Diabetes in Children and Adolescents
- Diabetes injury hazards
- Targeted blood Sugar Levels

CHAPTER 7

- Long-Term Strategies for Maintaining Blood Sugar Control

- medication and monitoring
- Ongoing Education and Support
- Strategies for Adjusting Your Plan

CONCLUSION

INTRODUCTION

A buildup of blood vessels and salt excretion by your kidneys are both lowered by excessive insulin, which also raises blood pressure.

Blood sugar levels that are consistently too high or too low can have various consequences on the body as a result of this I will be explaining the potential consequences of uncontrolled blood sugar levels and a remedy for it.

Blood sugar levels are a crucial variable with broad consequences for general health. It has an impact on exercise performance, hormone balance, brain function, diabetes management, and weight management. The key to sustaining general well-being and minimizing issues linked to both low and high blood sugar levels is maintaining a balanced blood sugar level through a healthy diet, frequent physical activity and appropriate medical management. It's critical to create a balanced, personal food plan for each kid or adolescent with diabetes. Your body releases cortisol and adrenaline, two stress chemicals that might raise blood sugar levels when you're under stress. By encouraging the liver to release glucose into the bloodstream, these hormones can raise blood sugar levels. Your sugar level can increase due to these factors and numerous others. Water is necessary for all cell functions, including those of the tissues that are healing. This affects the healing process. A healthy physique can help you manage your blood sugar levels more effectively. For those with diabetes, it's especially crucial to quench thirst and avoid dehydration through water consumption. To filter waste products, including glucose, the kidneys must work at their best, which can be maintained with adequate hydration.

The concentration of glucose in the bloodstream is referred to as blood sugar level, sometimes known as blood glucose level. For the body's cells to function properly,

glucose serves as their main source of energy. It is essential for overall health and is important for many physiological processes to maintain a healthy blood sugar level.

Regular blood glucose testing is the most important thing you can do to manage type 1 or type 2 diabetes is to exercise. You'll be able to watch what causes your numbers to climb or fall, such as eating different foods, taking your medication, or exercising. The ability to measure and monitor blood sugar fluctuations is made feasible by continuous glucose monitoring systems. Insights into patterns, trends, and variations are provided by CGM systems' near-real-time or real-time data on blood glucose levels. With the aid of this knowledge, patients and healthcare professionals may determine what causes blood sugar variability and alter their medication, diet, and lifestyle as appropriate. With this information, you can collaborate with your healthcare team to determine the optimal diabetes care strategy for you. Diabetes consequences such as heart attack, stroke, renal disease, blindness, and amputation can be delayed or avoided by making these choices. Be in hint with your healthcare provider at all times. In this book, you will also get strategies to know your blood sugar level without always rushing to the clinic or hospital for a check-up all the time.

CHAPTER 1

Blood Sugar Relevance to the Body

Blood sugar levels, also known as blood glucose levels, relate to the concentration of glucose (a form of sugar) in the bloodstream. Glucose is a main source of energy for the body's cells and is obtained through the breakdown of carbohydrates in the diet.

The body tightly regulates blood sugar levels to keep them within a certain range. Insulin, a pancreatic hormone, lowers blood sugar levels by promoting glucose uptake into cells. When blood sugar levels are excessively high, the pancreas produces insulin to increase glucose storage in the liver and muscle cells. When blood sugar levels fall too low, the pancreas secretes another hormone called glucagon, which stimulates the release of stored glucose into the bloodstream. The units used to measure blood sugar levels are often millimoles per liter (mmol/L) or milligrams per deciliter (mg/dL). Fasting blood sugar levels, which are calculated following an overnight fast, usually fall within the normal range of 70 to 100 mg/dL (3.9 to 5.6 mmol/L). The goal range may change, though, based on a person's age, health, and whether or not they have diabetes.

For overall health, steady blood sugar levels are essential. Hyperglycemia, or persistently high blood sugar levels, can be an indication of diabetes and, if untreated, can result in long-term consequences. Hypoglycemia, often known as low blood sugar, can cause symptoms like lightheadedness, confusion, and even unconsciousness. Blood sugar levels must be regularly monitored in people with diabetes, it's essential to ensure proper diabetes management.

The three major categories of blood sugar levels are:

1.**Random Blood Sugar:** Unaffected by fasting or meal scheduling, random blood sugar refers to the amount of glucose in the blood at any particular time. When someone is suffering signs of high or low blood sugar, it is frequently used in emergency settings. Although the appropriate range for blood sugar levels at random can vary, it is typically thought to be less than 200 mg/dL or 11.1 mmol/L.

For overall health and the avoidance of chronic diseases like diabetes, monitoring and maintaining blood sugar levels with a balanced diet, frequent exercise, and the right medicinal interventions are essential.

Blood sugar levels must be kept within healthy ranges for the body to produce energy, regulate metabolism, operate the brain, and be healthy overall. Blood sugar imbalances can significantly affect several biological processes and can play a role in the emergence of chronic diseases like diabetes. To keep it within a specific range, the blood's amount of glucose is tightly controlled. The body can suffer negative effects from blood sugar levels that are either too high or too low.

2.Hyperglycemia: a condition that is brought on by very high blood sugar levels. This frequently occurs in diabetics or when the body is unable to adequately manufacture or utilize the insulin that is produced. In these situations, too much glucose stays in the system, causing a variety of symptoms like increased thirst, frequent urination, weariness, and impaired vision. Organs, blood vessels, and nerves may eventually suffer harm from ongoing high blood sugar levels. Hypoglycemia, or low blood sugar, is the opposite and can happen as a result of excessive insulin release, insufficient calorie intake, or extended exercise without adequate nutrition.

3.Hypoglycemia: can cause sweating, confusion, dizziness, shakiness, and, in more extreme cases, seizures or loss of consciousness. Blood sugar levels must be raised right away to boost them and avoid issues. The central nervous system and the brain both depend on glucose for proper operation in addition to energy production. For maximum performance, the brain needs a consistent supply of glucose, which it uses intensively as its main energy source.

I will go over some of the major points about the importance of blood sugar in the body.

1.Energy Source: Glucose, which is produced when dietary carbs break down, travels through the bloodstream to all of the body's cells. To function, cells use glucose as fuel, which supplies energy for critical processes like muscular contraction, brain activity, and organ function.

2.Metabolism Control: Insulin, a hormone made by the pancreas, is essential for regulating blood sugar levels. After a meal, as blood sugar levels increase, insulin is secreted to encourage the uptake of glucose into cells and lower blood sugar levels. Limiting excessively high blood sugar levels (hyperglycemia) and encouraging the storage of extra glucose for future energy needs, aids in the regulation of metabolism.

3.Brain Function: Glucose serves as the primary energy source for the brain. For it to operate at its best, glucose must be available continuously. Hypoglycemia, or low blood sugar, can deprive the brain of enough energy, resulting in symptoms including disorientation, dizziness, and, in extreme cases, loss of consciousness. Blood sugar levels must be kept constant for proper brain function.

4.Diabetes Management: People with diabetes need to monitor and control their blood sugar levels more than anyone else. In type 1 diabetes, the pancreas does not produce insulin, but in type 2 diabetes, cells develop a resistance to insulin's actions. Regular blood sugar monitoring enables people to modify their food, medications, and lifestyle decisions to keep their blood sugar levels within a desired range. A healthy lifestyle and the prevention of complications are both aided by effective diabetes treatment.

5.Direct Health Effects: Extreme blood sugar levels may have direct health effects. Hyperglycemia, or high blood sugar, can cause symptoms like increased thirst, frequent urination, exhaustion, impaired vision, and, in more serious situations, diabetic ketoacidosis. Hypoglycemia, or low blood sugar, on the other hand, can result in symptoms including trembling, confusion, weakness, and, in severe cases, loss of consciousness. Maintaining blood sugar levels within a healthy range helps prevent these acute health issues.

Why did my blood sugar Spike?

Blood sugar spikes can occur for several reasons, especially in those with diabetes.

These typical causes of elevated blood sugar levels are listed below:

1.Carbohydrate intake: Eating a lot of carbs, particularly those with a high glycemic index (GI), can lead to a sharp rise in blood sugar levels. Sugary treats, refined grains, white bread, and sweetened beverages are examples of foods that might cause surges.

2.Insufficient insulin production or medication use: For diabetics, insufficient insulin production or inadequate medication use might cause increased blood sugar levels.

By making it easier for cells to absorb glucose, insulin aids in blood sugar regulation. Taking prescribed drugs as directed or skipping insulin doses might also cause an increase.

3.Insufficient exercise: Regular exercise can help lower blood sugar levels by assisting your body's use of glucose. Increased blood sugar levels may be caused by inactivity or protracted periods of inactivity.

4.Stress: When faced with stressful circumstances, the body releases stress chemicals like cortisol and adrenaline, which can raise blood sugar. To prevent spikes, stress can be managed through relaxation exercises or other coping mechanisms.

5.Disease or infection: The body releases more stress hormones when it is battling a disease or infection, which can raise blood sugar levels. When someone has a sickness, it's crucial to regularly monitor their blood sugar levels and modify their diabetes management.

When is the ideal time to check your blood sugar?

Depending on the goal of the test and the kind of diabetes you have, different times of day are appropriate for blood sugar checks

Here are a few general principles

1.The fasting blood sugar test (FBS): determines your blood sugar level the morning after an overnight fast. Before eating breakfast, it is typically done in the morning. Diabetes is frequently identified and tracked with FBS.

2.Postprandial blood sugar (PPBS): This examination gauges how your blood sugar levels change following a meal. It is usually carried out 1-2 hours after you begin eating. The PPBS tests your body's capacity to manage glucose after meals.

3.Random blood sugar (RBS): Regardless of when you last ate, this test can be performed at any time of the day. It offers a fast overview of your blood sugar level and is frequently used in emergencies or for quick examinations.

4.Blood sugar levels before exercise: If you regularly work out, you may need to check them before you begin. This will assist in ensuring that your blood sugar is within a safe level to avoid issues brought on by activity

5.Bedtime blood sugar:

It's important to check your blood sugar before bed, especially if you have diabetes. It assists in keeping track of your nighttime blood sugar control and identifying any treatment plan changes that may be necessary.

It's crucial to remember that the number and timing of blood sugar checks may change depending on

individual circumstances, including the type of diabetes, medication plan, general health, and advice from your healthcare professionals
To select the precise testing regimen that best meets your needs, it is important to speak with your doctor or a diabetes educator.

The Consequences of Raised and Decreased Blood Sugar Levels

The human body can suffer substantial effects from elevated or lowered blood sugar levels, sometimes referred to as **hyperglycemia** and **hypoglycemia**, respectively.

Hyperglycemia's negative effects include:

1.Diabetic ketoacidosis (DKA): A condition known as DKA can develop in people with diabetes when

blood sugar levels are continually high. It happens when the body doesn't produce enough insulin to turn glucose into energy, which forces the body to burn fat as fuel. This process results in the production of ketones, which cause an accumulation of acidic byproducts in the blood and may pose a life-threatening condition.

2.Organ Damage: Extended blood sugar elevations can harm several organs over time. Particularly at risk are the cardiovascular system, kidneys, eyes, and nerves. As a result, disorders such as diabetic nephropathy (kidney disease), retinopathy (eye

damage), neuropathy (nerve damage), and cardiovascular conditions may develop.

3.Increased Infection Risk: High blood sugar levels can weaken the immune system, making people more susceptible to infections. Bacterial and fungal infections, particularly in the urinary tract, skin, and respiratory system, are more likely in patients with poorly managed diabetes.

6.Health issues or medications: Corticosteroids, for example, might cause blood sugar levels to rise. Additional medical problems that might interfere with insulin production and cause spikes include hormonal imbalances (such as Cushing's syndrome) and illnesses that affect the pancreas.

7.Hormonal alterations: Changes in hormone levels, such as those that happen during menstruation or menopause, might affect blood sugar levels. During these times, some women might have blood sugar values that are higher.

8.Poor sleep: Lack of sleep or irregular sleep patterns can alter how well the body uses insulin and how quickly glucose is metabolized, thereby raising blood sugar levels.

The Consequences of Raised and Decreased Blood Sugar Levels

The human body can suffer substantial effects from elevated or lowered blood sugar levels, sometimes

referred to as hyperglycemia and hypoglycemia, respectively.

Hyperglycemia's negative effects include:

- **Diabetic ketoacidosis (DKA):** A condition known as DKA can develop in people with diabetes when blood sugar levels are continually high. It happens when the body doesn't produce enough insulin to turn glucose into energy, which forces the body to burn fat as fuel. This process results in the production of ketones, which cause an accumulation of acidic byproducts in the blood and may pose a life-threatening condition.

- **Organ Damage:** Extended blood sugar elevations can harm several organs over time. Particularly at risk are the cardiovascular system, kidneys, eyes, and nerves. As a result, disorders such as diabetic nephropathy (kidney disease), retinopathy (eye damage), neuropathy (nerve damage), and cardiovascular conditions may develop.

- **Increased Infection Risk:** High blood sugar levels can weaken the immune system, making people more susceptible to infections. Bacterial and fungal infections, particularly in the urinary tract, skin, and respiratory system, are more likely in patients with poorly managed diabetes.

- **Diabetic Coma:** If untreated, extremely high blood sugar levels might result in a diabetic coma. This is a life-threatening situation that necessitates immediate medical care intervention. It can happen in diabetics who have significant insulin shortages or consequences like DKA.

Effects of Low Blood Sugar Levels (Hypoglycemia)

1. Neurological Effects: When blood sugar levels go too low, the brain may not receive enough glucose to operate correctly. This can cause a variety of neurological symptoms such as confusion, difficulty concentrating, dizziness, migraines, mood swings, and, in severe cases, seizures.

2.Weakness and exhaustion: Hypoglycemia can cause a general feeling of weakness and exhaustion. Without enough glucose, the body's energy levels drop, impacting both physical and mental performance.

3.Anxiety and Irritability: Low blood sugar levels can cause feelings of anxiety, irritability, and nervousness. These symptoms may be accompanied by sweating, shaking, and an elevated heart rate.

4.Impaired Judgment and Coordination: Hypoglycemia has been shown to impair cognitive function, including judgment, decision-making, and coordination. This can influence daily tasks and increase the likelihood of an accident, particularly when driving or operating machinery.

5.Severe Hypoglycemia: Hypoglycemia can escalate to severe levels if left untreated, resulting in loss of consciousness or convulsions. This is a medical emergency that necessitates prompt treatment, such as the administration of glucose or glucagon.

It's necessary to remember that both high and low blood sugar levels can have different effects on a person's overall health, the length and severity of their disease, and other factors. Blood sugar levels must be managed and under control to avoid long-term difficulties and minimize any potential side effects related to these disorders.

To set suitable blood sugar goals and create a customized treatment strategy, diabetics should consult with medical professionals frequently.

Recognizing the terms (insulin, fructose, and glucose)

Most people mistakenly and interchangeably use these terms; I will enlighten you as to their proper definitions.

Glucose

The main source of energy for the body's cells is Glucose, a kind of sugar. Because it is a monosaccharide, it is a simple sugar molecule. Numerous body processes, such as cell metabolism, muscular contraction, and brain function, depend on glucose. Foods including fruits, vegetables, grains,

and sweetened items often include it. Hormones like insulin and glucagon control glucose in the body to keep blood sugar levels steady.

Fructose

Another form of sugar is Fructose, sometimes referred to as fruit sugar. Although it is a monosaccharide like glucose, its chemical makeup is distinct. Natural sources of fructose include honey, fruits, and vegetables.

Insulin

Many processed foods The pancreas releases insulin into the bloodstream in response to rising blood sugar levels.

Glucose can enter cells using insulin as a "key" and then be deployed as energy or saved for later use. Additionally, insulin aids in the storage of extra glucose as glycogen in the muscles and liver. Diabetes, a disorder marked by elevated blood sugar levels, can be brought on by insufficient insulin synthesis or impaired insulin activity.

This suggests that fructose is a different sort of sugar that is typically present in fruits and sweeteners, glucose is just sugar and the body's main source of energy, and insulin is a hormone that controls blood sugar levels by promoting the uptake and storage of glucose in cells and beverages also use it as a sweetener.

Fructose has a higher level of sweetness than glucose. Fructose is generally well tolerated by the body when taken in moderation from entire fruits. However, high-fructose corn syrup and other additional fructose intake have been associated with diseases like obesity and metabolic problems.

The pancreas, and more specifically the beta cells in the islets of Langerhans, produce the hormone insulin. It is essential for controlling blood sugar levels. When we eat carbs like glucose or fructose, the digestive system converts them into glucose molecules.

marked by elevated blood sugar levels, can be brought on by insufficient insulin synthesis or impaired insulin activity.

The following are insulin's main functions:

1.Glucose uptake: Insulin encourages cells to take up glucose, especially in muscle and fat tissue. The amount of glucose in the bloodstream is decreased because it improves the transit of glucose into these cells.

2.Glycogen synthesis: Insulin promotes the transformation of extra glucose into glycogen, a type of glucose that is stored in the body. The liver and muscle tissues store glycogen, which can later be converted into glucose as required.

Insulin inhibits the process known as gluconeogenesis, which causes the liver to produce less glucose. This aids in limiting the bloodstream's discharge of too much glucose.

3.Lipid synthesis: Insulin encourages the production of fatty acids and their storage in adipose tissue as triglycerides. Additionally, it prevents lipolysis, the process of breaking down fat reserves.

4.Protein synthesis: Insulin promotes the production of proteins and prevents their breakdown in a variety of tissues, aiding in the development and upkeep of bodily tissues.

CHAPTER 2

Glucagon

This is When blood glucose levels are low, such as during fasting or exercise, glucagon is generated and released by the pancreatic alpha cells. By triggering enzymes that release glucose from storage, it mostly raises blood sugar levels. The main functions of glucagon are as follows:

1.Glycogenolysis: Glucagon encourages the conversion of liver glycogen stores to glucose. The release of glucose into the bloodstream during this the procedure, known as glycogenolysis, raises blood sugar levels.

2.Gluconeogenesis: The creation of glucose from non-carbohydrate sources, such as amino acids and glycerol, is stimulated by glucagon. When nutritional sources of glucose are scarce, this aids in raising blood sugar levels.

3.Lipolysis: Glucagon promotes the breakdown of fats that have been accumulated in adipose tissue (lipolysis). The fatty acids from the released state can be used as an alternative energy source, sparing glucose for the brain and other tissues.

Ketogenesis: Under specific conditions, glucagon can encourage the production of ketone bodies from fatty acids. This happens when someone is fasting for a long time or when they have uncontrolled diabetes.

A careful balance between insulin and glucagon keeps blood sugar levels within a specific range. Insulin is released after a meal when blood sugar levels increase to help with carbohydrate absorption and storage. In contrast, glucagon is released when blood sugar levels drop to encourage the release of glucose that has been stored and to stimulate the creation of new glucose.

This dynamic interaction contributes to maintaining a steady supply of glucose for the body's energy generation.

The body's ability to use glucose and respond to insulin is known as insulin sensitivity. It is essential for preserving healthy metabolic function and regular blood sugar levels. People with high insulin sensitivity have cells that respond to insulin effectively and efficiently, allowing for the right uptake and utilization of glucose. This promotes steady blood sugar levels and prevents a significant accumulation of glucose in the blood.

Contrarily, persons with low insulin sensitivity, also known as insulin resistance, have decreased cell reactivity to insulin. As a result, blood sugar levels rise because the cells have a hard time absorbing glucose from the bloodstream. The pancreas generates more insulin as a retaliatory measure, raising blood levels of the hormone.

Conditions like type 2 diabetes, obesity, metabolic syndrome, and polycystic ovarian syndrome (PCOS) are frequently linked to insulin resistance. Genetics, lifestyle decisions (such as inactivity and bad food), and specific medical disorders might also have an impact.

Importance:

Insulin sensitivity is crucial for good health as it aids in controlling blood sugar levels and guards against the emergence of insulin resistance, a risk factor for type 2 diabetes. High blood sugar levels can be avoided by having cells that are effectively able to absorb glucose from the bloodstream.

Factors influencing insulin sensitivity

It's critical to keep in mind that these variables might interact and that there are many individual differences. Regardless of the specific causes, living a healthy lifestyle with regular exercise, a balanced diet, stress management, and enough sleep will help increase insulin sensitivity. Due to a genetic tendency, some people naturally have higher or lower insulin sensitivity

The factors influencing insulin are as follows.

1.Genetics: An individual's genetic makeup influences insulin sensitivity at birth. Some persons may be more or less sensitive to insulin due to genetic predisposition.

2.Body composition: Insulin sensitivity can be impacted by body fat percentage and distribution. Having too much body fat, especially visceral fat (fat around the organs), is linked to having less sensitive insulin receptors.

3.Drugs: Several drugs, including several HIV drugs, antipsychotics, and glucocorticoids (steroids), can impair insulin sensitivity and raise the risk of insulin resistance.

4.Chronic Inflammation: Insulin resistance can be exacerbated by inflammatory diseases, including obesity or persistent infections. Insulin sensitivity can be hampered by inflammation, which can interfere with normal insulin signaling pathways.

5.Sleep habit: Insufficient or poor-quality slumber has been linked to lowered insulin sensitivity. Lack of sleep has an impact on glucose metabolism and the body's hormonal balance.

6. Diet: The kind and quality of the diet might impact how sensitive the body is to insulin. Over time, a high diet of refined carbs, sweet foods, and drinks can cause insulin resistance.

Diets high in fiber, whole grains, fruits, vegetables, and lean proteins, on the other hand, have been linked to better insulin sensitivity.

1.Impacts of insulin sensitivity:
A good insulin response has various advantageous effects on health. It aids weight management, improves cardiovascular health, and improves overall metabolic function while lowering the chance of developing type 2 diabetes.

2.Insulin resistance: Insulin resistance can develop when insulin sensitivity decreases. This syndrome causes greater blood levels of insulin because the body's cells are less receptive to its actions. Metabolic syndrome is characterized by insulin resistance, which raises the risk of type 2 diabetes, obesity, heart disease, and other metabolic diseases.

3.Improved insulin sensitivity can be attained by making several lifestyle changes. Regular exercise,

maintaining a healthy weight, eating a balanced diet high in whole foods, cutting back on processed carbohydrates, managing portion sizes, managing stress levels, getting enough sleep, and thinking about intermittent fasting or time-restricted eating are a few of them. These techniques can improve insulin sensitivity and lower the chance of developing insulin resistance.

4.Monitoring insulin sensitivity:

The homeostatic model assessment of insulin resistance (HOMA-IR) and the oral glucose tolerance test (OGTT) are two common laboratory tests used to detect insulin sensitivity. These examinations measure how well the body manages insulin and glucose.

These tests, however, might not always be carried out on healthy people because they are typically done in clinical settings.

Does hypoglycemia resolve by itself?

Managing Hypoglycemia: Some Advice

Depending on the underlying reason and severity of the problem, hypoglycemia, or low blood sugar, can occasionally go away on its own. Hypoglycemia is frequently a symptom of an underlying medical issue, such as diabetes or certain hormone imbalances, and treating the underlying problem can help with hypoglycemia's symptoms.

When the triggering factor, such as excessive alcohol intake or an irregular eating pattern, is handled, hypoglycemia that was brought on by that specific incident may go away.

Consuming foods or beverages high in glucose, for instance, can help increase blood sugar levels and reduce hypoglycemia symptoms.

It's crucial to remember that persistent or recurring hypoglycemia may necessitate medical attention and continuing therapy. It is advised that you speak with a healthcare provider if you have recurrent episodes of hypoglycemia to receive an accurate diagnosis and a suitable treatment plan. To treat and prevent hypoglycemia episodes, they can suggest lifestyle modifications, medication modifications (if necessary), or other measures.

How eating food in the right order will help you lose weight

There is no scientific foundation for the idea that eating certain foods in a certain order will result in uncomplicated weight loss. While the order in which you consume your meals may have a slight effect on your fullness and digestion, it is not a major determinant of weight reduction.

When you eat fewer calories than your body requires, you experience weight loss because you have a calorie deficit. This can be accomplished in several ways, including cutting back on portion sizes, consuming foods that are high in nutrients, and exercising frequently.

"Food combining" diets frequently promote the idea of eating certain foods in a particular order to promote weight loss.

Water consumption: To stay hydrated and promote general health, drink plenty of water throughout the day.

Exercise or physical activity regularly can help you lose weight. In general, adopting a balanced and sustainable strategy for eating for weight loss is more efficient than focusing on the order of items. A balanced diet should contain a range of foods that are high in nutrients, such as fruits, vegetables, whole grains, lean meats, and healthy fats.

Eat mindfully, pay attention to your hunger and fullness cues, and eat slowly to prevent overeating.

Does weight loss affect blood sugar levels?

Yes, Particularly for people with diabetes or prediabetes, weight loss can significantly affect blood sugar levels.

Here is how losing weight may impact blood sugar levels:

1.Increased Insulin Sensitivity: Extra body weight, particularly belly fat, can cause insulin resistance, a condition where cells lose their sensitivity to insulin. An important hormone in controlling blood sugar levels is insulin. Elevated blood sugar levels occur when cells become resistant to insulin, making it harder for glucose to enter cells. Weight loss, particularly when accompanied by a healthy diet and exercise, can increase insulin sensitivity, facilitating the uptake of glucose into cells and resulting in a reduction in blood sugar levels.

2.Reduced HbA1c Levels: HbA1c is an indicator of the average blood sugar levels over the previous two to three months. HbA1c values can drop as a result of weight loss, indicating better blood sugar regulation. Maintaining lower HbA1c levels is crucial for people with diabetes as it lowers their risk of developing long-term consequences from their condition.

3.Reduction in Medications Needed: Some people with type 2 diabetes may be able to cut back on or stop taking their diabetes medications if they can achieve and maintain a healthy weight through lifestyle modifications like a balanced diet and frequent exercise.

Weight loss can help regulate blood sugar, necessitating prescription modifications. But before adjusting a medication's dosage, it's important to speak with a medical expert.

4.Better Overall Glycemic Control: Losing weight can result in improved overall glycemic control, which means that blood sugar levels stay more stable throughout the day. Less variation in blood sugar levels can be achieved by adopting a healthy lifestyle and lowering weight, which lowers the chance of developing hyperglycemia (high blood sugar) or hypoglycemia (low blood sugar).

Strategies of mindful eating and portion control

Maintaining a positive relationship with food and controlling portions can help with weight management.

some tactics that can be used.

1. Chew your meal thoroughly and savor every bite: Take your time, and enjoy the flavor, texture, and aroma of your food. This enables you to take full advantage of your meal and gives your brain enough time to recognize when you are full.

2. Use smaller plates and bowls: Choose smaller plates and bowls to give the impression that the dish is fuller. This can aid in portion management and assist in stopping overeating.

3. Attend to your body's signals of hunger and fullness: Eat only when you are hungry by paying attention to your body. Eat till you are satisfied without going overboard. to abstain from eating when under boredom, stress, or other emotional stressors

.

4. Prepare your meals in advance by portioning them out; otherwise, you'll end yourself eating straight from a bag or container. This helps you become more conscious of how much you're eating and discourages thoughtless munching.

5. Put a lot of vegetables on your plate: Make eating a lot of vegetables a priority. They make you feel satisfied for longer and have a high fiber content, which helps you naturally regulate portion sizes.

6. Engage in mindful snacking by selecting wholesome foods and paying attention to serving portions. Put a tiny piece in a bowl or on a plate rather than eating straight from the bag. By doing this, mindless eating is avoided.

7. Limit distractions: Limit your use of phones, televisions, and other electronic devices while you're eating. You may concentrate on the sensory experience of eating when you pay close attention to your meal, which also helps you avoid overeating.

8. Keep a food diary: Keeping track of your meals and snacks will help you become more mindful of portion sizes as well as see any patterns or reasons why you tend to overeat. Additionally, it can assist you in changing your eating patterns.

9.Educate yourself on portion proportions for various food groups and practice portion management tactics. Make use of visual cues, such as comparing a serving size to commonplace items (a deck of cards, for example, for meat). Even without access to measuring instruments, this can help you control and estimate portion amounts.

10. Seek assistance: Take into account getting assistance from a qualified dietician or signing up for a support group that emphasizes mindful eating and portion control. They can offer direction, responsibility, and additional tactics that cater to your unique needs.

It takes time and effort to develop long-lasting habits like mindful eating and portion control. Be kind to yourself and concentrate on modifying your eating habits in a sustainable, progressive manner.

CHAPTER 3

For Stable Blood Glucose: Diet and Nutrition

NUTRITION

The process through which living things acquire and use food to sustain their development, growth, and general health is referred to as nutrition. Intake, digestion, absorption, transport, metabolism, and excretion of nutrients from food are all included.

The body needs nutrients for effective operation, which are elements that are present in the diet.

Carbohydrates, lipids, proteins, vitamins, minerals, and water are the six main categories of nutrients.

To ensure optimal intake of these nutrients, it is essential to follow a balanced diet that consists of a variety of foods from various food categories. Malnutrition, obesity, and chronic illnesses including cardiovascular disease, diabetes, and some types of cancer can all be caused by poor nutrition, in addition to other health issues.

DIET

The kinds of food and beverages that an individual or a group of people consumes are referred to as their diet. It can also be used to describe a particular eating regimen that is followed for a variety of purposes, including maintaining or enhancing

general health, attaining weight loss or gain objectives, managing particular medical problems, or accommodating dietary limitations. Before making large dietary changes.

it is advised to speak with a healthcare provider or trained dietitian. Any particular diet should be customized to each person's needs and interests. Depending on cultural, regional, and individual preferences, dietary habits might differ significantly.

Diets that are often used include:

1. **Balanced Diet:** Consuming a range of foods from several food groups, including fruits, vegetables, whole grains, and lean meats, constitutes a balanced diet

2. **The Mediterranean diet**: This is based on the customary eating patterns of the inhabitants of the nations that border the Mediterranean Sea. It places a focus on plant-based foods such as fruits, vegetables, whole grains, legumes, nuts, and olive

oil while also including small amounts of dairy, fish, and fowl.

3. Low-Carb Diet: Diets that are low in carbohydrates, such as those that exclude grains, starchy vegetables, and sugary meals, are not recommended. Usually, they promote eating more protein and fat. The ketogenic diet, the Atkins diet, and the South Beach diet are all well-known low-carb eating plans

.

4. Vegan diet: A vegan diet forgoes any goods derived from animals, including dairy, eggs, honey, fish, meat, and poultry. It consists mostly of plant-based foods such as fruits, vegetables, grains, legumes, nuts, and seeds. For ethical, environmental, or health reasons, vegans may opt for this diet.

5. Paleo Diet: The paleo diet aims to resemble our predecessors' diets during the Paleolithic period. It excludes grains, legumes, dairy, and processed foods in favor of unprocessed foods including lean meats, fish, fruits, vegetables, nuts, and seeds.

6. Gluten-Free Diet: A gluten-free diet excludes gluten, a protein that is present in various cereals, including rye, barley, and wheat. For anyone with celiac disease or non-celiac gluten sensitivity, this diet is crucial.

Nutrition for Blood Glucose Stability

Particularly for people with diabetes or those who want to avoid blood sugar fluctuations, maintaining stable blood glucose levels is important for overall health.

To help maintain blood sugar levels, the following dietary and nutritional suggestions are provided:

1.Eat a Balanced Diet: Put your attention on having a balanced diet that consists of a variety of complex carbs, lean proteins, healthy fats, and high-fiber foods. By reducing the rate at which glucose is absorbed into the system, this method helps prevent sharp increases in blood sugar levels.

Select foods with a low glycemic index (GI): The glycemic index gauges how rapidly foods high in carbohydrates boost blood sugar levels. Low GI

foods are absorbed more gradually and affect blood sugar levels less. Include things like legumes, non-starchy veggies, most fruits, and whole grains (like quinoa and brown rice).

Keep an eye on your carb intake because they have the most effect on your blood sugar levels. Counting carbohydrates and controlling portions can be useful. To determine the proper carbohydrate consumption for your unique requirements, think about working with a certified dietitian who specializes in diabetes management.

2.Include Lean Proteins: Protein-rich foods including lean meats, poultry, fish, eggs, tofu, lentils, and low-fat dairy products can aid slow carbohydrate digestion, avoiding blood sugar spikes.

Include sources of healthy fats such as avocados, nuts, seeds, olive oil, and fatty fish (e.g., salmon, sardines) in your diet. These fats supply critical nutrients and enhance satiety, which aids in blood sugar control and appetite management.

- **Increase Fiber Intake:** By slowing digestion and fostering a steady release of glucose into the bloodstream, high-fiber foods can help regulate blood sugar levels. Soluble fiber sources such as oats, barley, legumes, fruits, and vegetables should be included.

- **Avoid Sugary** and Refined Meals: Reduce or eliminate your intake of sugary beverages, processed meals, and refined grains (white rice).

- **Keep Hydrated:** To stay properly hydrated, sip lots of water throughout the day. Drinks with added sugar should be restricted or avoided as they might cause rapid blood sugar rises.

- **To limit your overall calorie consumption,** practice portion control by being aware of meal sizes. Even healthful meals, if ingested in excess, can affect blood sugar levels.

- **Regular Meal Timing:** Create a regular eating routine and refrain from skipping meals. Meal schedule consistency can help control blood sugar levels and lessen excessive changes.

As individual dietary needs can vary, it's vital to speak with a registered dietitian or other healthcare provider who can offer tailored advice based on your unique health situation and goals.

Some varieties of foods may drop your blood sugar, but some may do it more quickly than others.
Although other factors that affect blood sugar control include body weight, activity, stress, and heredity, maintaining a balanced diet is essential for blood sugar control (1 Trusted Source, 2 Trusted Source).

Even though some foods, such as those that are high in added sugar and refined carbohydrates, might cause blood sugar oscillations, other foods can improve blood sugar management while fostering health.

The 17 Healthiest Foods for Blood Sugar Control

- Broccoli
- Seafood
- Pumpkin
- Nuts
- Flaxseed
- Beans
- Fermented food
- the chia seed
- Kale
- Berries
- Avocados
- Oats
- Citrus
- Azzi

- Kefir

- Eggs

- Apples

1. Broccoli: Research on animals, in test tubes, and a few human studies have demonstrated that sulforaphane-rich broccoli extract has strong anti-diabetic benefits, improving insulin sensitivity and lowering blood sugar and oxidative stress indicators.

Glucosinolates like glucoraphanin are concentrated in broccoli sprouts. When taken as a supplement in the form of a powder or extract, these substances may assist persons with type 2 diabetes in improving their insulin sensitivity and lowering their blood sugar levels.

2. Seafood

Seafood generally has a modest impact on blood sugar levels due to its low carbohydrate content.

Rich in protein and healthy fats, it is a beneficial choice for individuals managing blood sugar. However, some preparations, such as fried or sweet sauces, might elevate levels.

Because of their low calorie and carbohydrate content, kimchi and sauerkraut can both be part of a healthy diet for blood sugar control. However, additional sugars and other foods that may raise the glycemic load must be avoided. Furthermore, because individual reactions to these foods can vary, it is recommended that you monitor your blood sugar levels and speak with a healthcare professional.

3. Consistent meals and snacks: Maintain consistent meal schedules and prevent extended gaps between meals. This helps to keep blood glucose levels stable. If necessary, include healthy snacks between meals to keep blood sugar levels stable

4. Hydration: Drink lots of water all day long to stay hydrated. Avoid drinking too much coffee and sugary drinks because they can raise blood sugar levels.

5. Glycemic index: Get to know the glycemic index (GI) of various foods. Foods with a lower GI value typically affect blood sugar levels more gently. Increase your consumption of low- to medium-GI

meals, but keep in mind that portion sizes still matter.

6. Monitor and adjust: Keep a close eye on your blood sugar levels and seek advice from a certified dietician or healthcare provider. They can assist you in making changes to your diet and nutrition plan and offer specialized advice based on your unique needs.

Keep in mind that it's essential to customize nutritional recommendations depending on your unique health requirements and situations. Working with a licensed dietician or healthcare provider can offer you individualized advice that is suited to your needs.

Meal planning is a great way to ensure balanced nutrition, organize your meals in advance, save time, and reduce food waste. Here are some guidelines for meal preparation and some sample menus:

1. Evaluate your dietary objectives: Take into account your nutritional requirements, including calorie consumption, the ratio of carbs to proteins and fats, and any particular dietary preferences or limits.

2. Plan your meals: Allocate time each week to make a meal plan. Make a general sketch of what you want to eat after selecting how many meals you want to schedule (breakfast, lunch, supper, and snacks).

3. Balance your plate: Aim for meals that are well-balanced and contain a variety of lean proteins, whole grains, healthy fats, and a lot of fruits and vegetables. This keeps you full and helps give you the necessary nutrients.

4. Make use of seasonal produce: Include seasonal fruits and vegetables in your menu plan. They are frequently more flavorful, more nutrient-dense, and more inexpensive.

5. Create a shopping list based on your meal plan. List all the ingredients you'll need to buy. When you go grocery shopping, stick to your list to prevent making impulse buys.

6. Batch cooking and meal preparation: Think about preparing ingredients ahead of time or batch cooking huge quantities of some meals. This can save time on hectic weekdays and make it simpler to adhere to your schedule.

7. Flexibility and variety: To keep things interesting, mix up the ingredients and flavors in your meals. Your strategy should have a certain amount of freedom to account for adjustments or unplanned events.

Let's look at an example of a meal plan for the day :

Breakfast:

- Avocado spread over whole-wheat bread - Fresh fruit salad

Greek yogurt and berries are healthy snacks.

Lunch: consists of grilled chicken breast, quinoa, and roasted veggies (zucchini, carrots, and broccoli). A mixed green salad with cherry tomatoes and balsamic vinaigrette completes the meal.

Snack:

Carrot sticks and hummus

Dinner:

consist of steamed asparagus, baked salmon with lemon and dill, brown rice pilaf, and a side salad with feta cheese, mixed greens, and cucumber.

Snacking on apple slices with almond butter

Keep in mind that this is only one example and that you can modify your meal plan to suit your tastes and nutritional needs. You'll discover the meal-planning strategy that works best for you with experience and testing.

Carbohydrates: Types, Glycemic Index, and Blood Glucose Influence.

Along with proteins and fats, carbohydrates are one of the three major macronutrients in meals. They are the body's major source of energy and are essential for maintaining healthy biological functions. Different types of carbohydrates can affect blood glucose levels differently, depending on their composition and glycemic index, among other things.

Carbohydrate varieties: Based on their chemical structure, carbohydrates can be divided into three primary categories:

1. Simple carbs: Quickly absorbed by the body, these carbs are composed of one or two sugar units. Examples include glucose, fructose, which is present in fruits, and lactose, which is present in milk.

2. Complex Carbohydrates: These carbohydrates require more time to digest and are made up of lengthy chains of sugar molecules. Examples include the starches in legumes, root vegetables, and grains.

3. Dietary fiber: Fiber is a kind of carbohydrate that the body is unable to break down. It typically makes it through the digestive system undamaged.

Glycemic Index (GI):

The glycemic index is a measure that assigns a blood glucose level-raising capability to each carbohydrate in comparison to a reference food, often glucose or white bread. The GI is a gauge of how quickly the body digests and absorbs a certain carbohydrate. High GI carbohydrates are broken down and absorbed more quickly, leading to a more pronounced rise in blood sugar levels.

Simple carbs like white bread, white rice, and sugary snacks are frequently foods with a high GI. Commonly, complex carbohydrates or foods abundant in fiber, like whole grains, fruits, and vegetables, have a low GI. Since low GI meals take

longer to digest, there is a slower and more gradual increase in blood sugar levels.

Blood Glucose Influence: Consuming carbs, especially those with a high GI, can have a big effect on blood sugar levels. High GI carbohydrates are promptly converted into glucose and absorbed into circulation after consumption. This results in a sharp rise in blood glucose levels, which prompts the pancreas to produce more insulin to control blood sugar levels.

A slower and more controlled release of glucose into the bloodstream occurs as a result of the slower digestion of low GI carbohydrates. This promotes more consistent blood glucose levels and offers a constant supply of energy for a longer amount of time.

For people with illnesses like diabetes, controlling blood glucose levels is very crucial. They might need to be careful of their carbohydrate intake, choose carbohydrates with a low GI, and balance their consumption with other nutrients to maintain stable blood sugar levels. The total amount and kind of carbohydrates ingested, as well as individual aspects like metabolism and activity level, can all affect blood glucose responses. This is vital to keep in mind. Personal advice on controlling carbohydrate intake and blood glucose levels can be obtained by speaking with a healthcare provider or qualified dietitian.

Carbohydrate Counting

People with diabetes can control their blood sugar levels by measuring carbohydrates. It entails monitoring the number of carbs ingested throughout the day at meals and snacks.

One of the nutrients that has the most influence on blood sugar levels is carbohydrates. As glucose enters the bloodstream as a result of the breakdown of carbs, blood sugar levels rise. Diabetes sufferers can better manage their blood sugar levels by keeping an eye on and restricting their carbohydrate intake.

The fundamental procedures for carbohydrate counting are as follows:

1.Recognizing the sources of carbohydrates: Find out which foods are high in carbs. Grain products, bread, rice, pasta, starchy fruits and vegetables, dairy products, legumes, and sweets are included in this category. It's crucial to remember that different foods contain varying types and amounts of carbs.

2. Determining serving sizes: Become familiar with the typical serving amounts for various foods that include carbohydrates. You can do this by consulting food databases, nutrition labels, or measuring equipment.

3. Tracking carbohydrate grams: Keep a log of how many grams of carbohydrates you ingest overall at each meal and snack. You can do this manually, with the aid of smartphone apps, or online using tools made specifically for counting carbohydrates.

4. Setting personal carbohydrate goals: Consult a certified dietitian or healthcare professional to establish an appropriate daily carbohydrate goal based on variables like age, weight, amount of activity, and diabetes control strategy.

5. Changing the dosage of insulin or other medications: People who take insulin or specific diabetes medications may need to change their dosages to correspond to the number of carbohydrates they ingest. A healthcare expert should be consulted before doing this.

6. Regularly check blood sugar levels: to determine how much of an influence eating carbohydrates has on glycemic management. Adjusting medicine and carbohydrate counts can be made more precise with the use of this information.

People with diabetes may make educated decisions about their dietary consumption thanks to carbohydrate counting, which gives meal planning flexibility.

It gives individuals the ability to match their carbohydrate consumption with drug or insulin dosages to reach desired blood sugar levels. For people who use intense insulin therapy or who receive many daily insulin injections, carbohydrate counting is often advised.

The outcome of using carbohydrate counting

The main benefit of carbohydrate counting for diabetics is better blood sugar regulation. People can better control their blood sugar levels and lower their risk of developing hyperglycemia (high blood sugar) or hypoglycemia by monitoring and limiting their carbohydrate consumption.

The advantages and outcomes of carb counting are as follows:

1. Blood sugar control: Diabetes sufferers who calculate their carbohydrates are better able to comprehend how their blood sugar levels are directly affected by carbohydrates.

They can keep blood glucose levels more consistently steady throughout the day by correctly tracking carbohydrate intake and adjusting insulin or prescription doses accordingly.

2. Flexibility in meal planning and carbohydrate counting: Meal planning can be flexible when using carbohydrate counting. People can do this and yet efficiently control their blood sugar levels while eating a range of meals. Without entirely restricting any one food group, people who are skilled at carb counting can make educated decisions about the items they eat and the portions they eat.

3. Individualized approach: Carbohydrate counting considers a person's individual needs, including age, weight, amount of exercise, and diabetes control

strategy. The carbohydrate objectives are adapted to the individual's particular circumstances in this individualized strategy, which results in better blood sugar control.

4. Better insulin or medication management: Counting carbohydrates enables people to modify their insulin or medication doses by the number of carbohydrates consumed. Because of this, carbohydrate intake and insulin response can be better timed, resulting in more accurate blood sugar control.

5. Increased self-awareness and empowerment: Counting carbohydrates encourages people to be more conscientious of their dietary choices and serving sizes. As a result, one's self-awareness and

a sense of control over managing their diabetes are strengthened. It encourages a better understanding of how various foods affect blood sugar levels.

6. Complications are prevented: Consistently keeping blood sugar levels within the target range can help lower the risk of long-term complications

of diabetes, including heart disease, nerve damage, kidney illness, and eye issues.

Carbohydrate counting is just one aspect of diabetes management. I will always advise you to keep in touch with your health advice.

CHAPTER 4

Microbiome

Microbiome

A living organism's surface and internal microorganisms, such as bacteria, viruses, fungi, and other microbes, collectively make up its microbiome. These microbes create intricate and varied communities in the skin, mouth, gut, and reproductive organs, among other areas of the body. Numerous elements, including genetics, diet, lifestyle, drugs, and environmental exposures, have an impact on the microbiome's composition. Dysbiosis, or disruptions or imbalances in the microbiome, has been linked to several illnesses, such as inflammatory bowel disease, obesity, diabetes, allergies, and mental health issues.

The human microbiome is critical to sustaining general health and carrying out necessary tasks. It interacts with the host organism in a way that is advantageous to both parties. For instance, the gut microbiome aids in nutritional digestion and absorption, manufactures specific vitamins, and contributes to the growth and operation of the immune system. The metabolism, mental health, immune responses, and other elements of human health are thought to be impacted by it.

The term **"gut microbiome"** describes the variety of microbes that live in our gastrointestinal system,

including bacteria, viruses, fungi, and other microbes. The gut microbiota is critical for maintaining several elements of our health, including the control of blood sugar, according to recent research.

The composition of the gut microbiome has been linked in several studies to the emergence of diseases like type 2 diabetes and insulin resistance. It has been noted that people with type 2 diabetes typically have a distinct composition of the gut microbiota than people without the disease. These variations include changes in the prevalence of particular bacterial species or groupings.

Several theories explain how the gut plants affect blood sugar levels:
1. Dietary fiber fermentation: The gut microbiota can break down dietary fiber that humans are unable

to digest, resulting in the production of short-chain fatty acids (SCFAs) as a consequence. SCFAs, like butyrate, have been demonstrated to promote glucose metabolism and improve insulin sensitivity, which helps control blood sugar levels.

2. Bile acid metabolism: Bile acids are involved in glucose regulation and fat digestion, and their metabolism is also influenced by the gut flora. Blood sugar management may be impacted by changes in bile acid metabolism caused by gut bacteria.

3. Inflammation and Gut Barrier Function: Imbalances in the composition of the gut microbiome may increase gut permeability and result in persistent low-grade inflammation. This inflammation may obstruct insulin signaling, increase insulin resistance, and eventually impair blood sugar regulation.

4. Gut Hormone Regulation: The production and secretion of hormones related to appetite regulation, such as glucagon-like peptide-1 (GLP-1) and peptide YY (PYY), can be affected by the gut microbiota. These hormones influence blood sugar levels and general metabolic health by contributing to satiety and glucose homeostasis.

Researchers are looking into interventions to modify the gut microbiota for medicinal purposes, given the possible impact of the gut microbiome on blood sugar management.

Investigated tactics comprise the following:

1. Probiotics and prebiotics: Probiotics are beneficial living bacteria that can be taken to alter the composition of the gut microbiome. Prebiotics are dietary fibers that provide the good bacteria in the gut with sustenance. The ability of probiotics and prebiotics to enhance insulin sensitivity and blood sugar regulation is currently being researched.

2. Fecal Microbiota Transplantation (FMT): FMT involves giving a recipient feces that contain a healthy gut microbiome from a donor. This method has shown promise in the treatment of a few gastrointestinal disorders, and it is also being

investigated for its potential to enhance metabolic health, including blood sugar management.

3. Dietary Changes: Diet has a significant impact on the gut flora. Certain dietary patterns, such as a high-fiber diet or certain plant-based diets, have been linked to a more favorable gut microbiota composition and better blood sugar control.

Obtaining Macronutrient Balance with Protein and Fat

What is a macronutrient?

A macronutrient is a type of food that the body needs in relatively significant amounts to maintain several physiological processes and give energy. Water, vitamins, and minerals should not be left out of the list of the three macronutrients below because they each play a different role in the growth and development of the human body. However, for the sake of this discussion, I will focus on attaining a macronutrient balance with proteins and fats.

Definitions of the three primary macronutrients

1. Carbohydrates: The body uses carbohydrates as its primary energy source. They are converted into glucose, which the cells use as fuel. Foods like grains, fruits, vegetables, and legumes contain carbohydrates.

2. Proteins: Proteins are necessary for the development, maintenance, and repair of all body tissues. They are made up of amino acids, which serve as the foundation for proteins. Meat, poultry, fish, eggs, dairy products, legumes, and nuts are all excellent sources of protein.

3. Fats: Fats are essential for supplying energy, acting as insulation, and safeguarding organs. Monounsaturated and polyunsaturated fats, which

may be found in nuts, seeds, avocados, and fatty fish, are thought to be healthier than saturated and trans fats, which can be found in fried foods, processed snacks, and some animal products, even though fats are a concentrated source of calories.

Proteins

Amino acids are the building blocks of life. Amino acids are molecules used by all living things to make proteins They are fundamental macronutrients needed by the body for several processes. Proteins are essential for the development, maintenance, and repair of tissues as well as for the synthesis of hormones, enzymes, and antibodies.

The 20 different types of amino acids that can be combined in various ways to create a large range of

proteins are the building blocks of proteins. Essential amino acids and non-essential amino acids are the two groups into which these amino acids fall. Both animal and plant-based sources contain proteins. Meat, poultry, fish, eggs, and dairy products are all examples of animal sources of protein. Legumes (beans, lentils, and chickpeas), soy products (tofu, tempeh), and nuts are all plant-based sources of protein

macronutrient balance with protein

To achieve a macronutrient balance with protein, you must make sure you eat enough of it in addition to other macronutrients, such as carbohydrates and fats, to satisfy your dietary demands.

The three main food groups that give us energy are known as macronutrients: protein, carbs, and fats. Building and mending tissues, making enzymes and hormones, and maintaining various biological activities all depend on protein.

The following factors should be taken into account to get a balanced macronutrient intake with protein:

1.Ascertain your protein requirements: The daily recommended consumption of protein varies based on age, sex, weight, level of physical activity, and general health. To determine the proper protein consumption for your individual needs, speak with a qualified dietitian or other medical expert.

2.Determine your protein sources: Include a range of high-quality protein sources in your diet, such as tofu, tempeh, seitan, eggs, dairy products (milk,

yogurt, cheese), legumes (beans, lentils, chickpeas), dairy products (milk, yogurt, cheese), dairy products (milk, yogurt, cheese), and dairy products (milk, yogurt, cheese). The necessary amino acids found in these sources are what make up protein's building blocks.

3. Combine protein with carbohydrates and fats: For a well-rounded macronutrient balance, it's vital to include carbohydrates and fats in your meals in addition to protein. Choose complex carbs like whole grains, fruits, vegetables, and legumes as well as healthy fats from sources like olive oil, avocados, nuts, and seeds.

4. Portion control: Keep track of your serving sizes to make sure you're getting the right ratio of macronutrients. Use recommended serving sizes as a guideline and adjust them according to your specific goals and needs

5. Spread out your protein consumption throughout the day: Instead of getting the majority of your protein from a single meal, spread it out evenly throughout the day. This strategy enhances the production of muscle protein while supplying a consistent stream of amino acids for a variety of biological processes.

6. Give meal planning some thought: Planning your meals and snacks can help you consume a variety of macronutrients. Aim to incorporate a supply of

protein, carbs, and fats in each meal and snack to ensure a balanced nutritional profile.

Fats

One of the three macronutrients, along with proteins and carbs, is fat. Although it has been stigmatized in the past, fat is an important component of a healthy diet and serves several vital purposes for the body. Focusing on ingesting healthy fats and keeping a balanced intake is crucial when acquiring macronutrients with fat.

Here are some sources of good fats:

1. Avocados: Monounsaturated fats, which are regarded as beneficial fats, are abundant in avocados. They are also a rich source of vitamins, fiber, and other important elements like potassium.

2. Nuts and seeds: Hemp, chia, flax, and walnut seeds are all fantastic sources of healthy fats. They also offer fiber, vitamins, minerals, and protein.

3. Fatty fish: Fish that are high in omega-3 fatty acids include trout, salmon, mackerel, and sardines.Omega-3 is an essential part of the diet and supplements like fish oil have been associated with several health benefits.

4. Extra virgin olive oil: is a main stay of Mediterranean cooking and is renowned for its monounsaturated fat content. It can be used in cooking, salad dressings, and as a bread dip.

5. Coconut oil includes medium-chain triglycerides (MCTs): a form of healthy fat despite being heavy in saturated fat. In moderation, it can be added to smoothies,baked products, and cooking.

6. Dark chocolate: Chocolate with a high cocoa content includes antioxidants and good fats. Choose products with less sugar added.

Fats are calorie-dense, you should take them in moderation and pay attention to portion sizes to maintain a balanced diet. Despite this, fat is still a crucial macronutrient

Should a diabetic avoid fats?

Although people with diabetes don't have to completely avoid fats, it's still necessary to pay attention to the kinds and amounts that are consumed. While some fats may be healthy, others, particularly when ingested in excess, may be harmful. Here are some recommendations for people with diabetes regarding their diet of fat:

1. Choose healthful fats: Pay special attention to consuming monounsaturated and polyunsaturated fats, which can improve insulin sensitivity and cardiovascular health. These fats may be found in foods like avocados, almonds, seeds, olive oil, fatty fish (including salmon, mackerel, and sardines), and flaxseeds.

2. Eat less saturated and trans fats: Saturated fats, which are found in large quantities in meat, dairy products, and butter, can raise cholesterol levels and raise your risk of heart disease. Since trans fats are exceedingly dangerous and are usually present in processed and fried foods, they should never be taken. Because trans fats are frequently present, carefully read food labels and avoid anything manufactured with partially hydrogenated oils.

3. Control portion sizes: Because fats are high in calories, it's important to keep portion proportions under control. To avoid taking too many calories, which can cause weight gain and disrupt blood sugar

homeostasis, even healthy fats should be consumed in moderation.

4. Include fats in a diet that includes carbohydrates, proteins, and other nutrients to keep it balanced. As a result of the slower glucose absorption, blood sugar levels may become more steady. For instance, eating fiber-rich carbs along with healthy fats might delay digestion and lessen blood sugar increases.

5. Tailored approach: It's necessary to work with a healthcare expert or registered dietitian who specializes in diabetes management to create a tailored meal plan that takes into account your unique needs, blood sugar control objectives, and general health state.

The appropriate ratio of protein to fat in your diet is crucial for general health and well-being. Both macronutrients have distinctive roles in the body as well as functions and advantages

Fiber's Essential Function in Blood Glucose Management

The management of blood sugar levels and the advancement of general health depend heavily on fiber. As a result, it passes through the digestive system mainly undigested because it is a form of carbohydrate that the body cannot digest. The two primary forms of fiber are soluble and insoluble, and both can help control blood sugar levels.

Water dissolves soluble fiber, which then congeals in the intestines to produce a gel-like material. The slowing down of carbohydrate digestion and absorption by this gel aids in reducing post-meal blood glucose rises. By lowering calorie intake, soluble fiber also encourages a sensation of fullness and can aid in weight control.

Insoluble fiber, on the other hand, bulks up the stool and aids in the promotion of regular bowel motions. While it has no direct effect on blood glucose levels, it can indirectly help with glucose control by decreasing nutrient absorption, particularly carbohydrate absorption, and reducing blood sugar spikes.

<u>Including enough fiber in the diet has various advantages for blood glucose management:</u>

1. **Blood sugar regulation:** Soluble fiber produces a gel that delays carbohydrate digestion and absorption, avoiding abrupt rises in blood glucose levels. This helps to maintain more consistent blood sugar levels over time.

2.**Improved insulin sensitivity:** According to research, a high-fiber diet may improve insulin sensitivity, which is critical for the body's capacity to use insulin effectively and regulate blood sugar levels.

3. **Lowering the risk of type 2 diabetes:** Diets high in fiber have been linked to a lower risk of acquiring type 2 diabetes. Fiber's capacity to improve blood sugar regulation and promote a healthy body weight is assumed to be the reason for this.

4.**Weight management:** Fiber-rich foods are more full, which can help control hunger and lower calorie intake. This can help with weight management because being overweight is a risk factor for type 2 diabetes and can impair blood glucose control.

Consuming a range of whole, unprocessed foods such as fruits, vegetables, legumes, whole grains, nuts, and seeds is recommended to improve fiber intake

. The American Dietetic Association advises a daily fiber consumption of 25 to 38 grams for people, however, individual needs may vary.

It's important to remember that if you have diabetes or any other medical condition, you should contact a healthcare expert or a qualified dietitian for individualized dietary recommendations. They can advise on fiber incorporation.

CHAPTER 5

Sleep Quality and its Impact on Blood Glucose Levels

Sleep quality can have a significant impact on blood glucose levels, especially for individuals with diabetes. Poor sleep or insufficient sleep can disrupt the body's hormonal balance and lead to imbalances in blood sugar control.

The following are some ways that blood sugar levels might be affected by the quality of sleep: Insufficient sleep has been related to insulin resistance, which occurs when the body's cells stop

responding positively to the effects of insulin. Higher blood glucose levels brought on by insulin resistance may contribute to the onset or progression of type 2 diabetes.

Cortisol levels: The stress hormone cortisol can be increased by sleep loss or poor sleep. Higher blood sugar levels can be caused by elevated cortisol levels, which prompt the liver to release more glucose into the blood.

controlling appetite: such as leptin and ghrelin, can become out of balance when people don't get enough sleep. This disruption may result in increased appetite, cravings for meals high in calories, and overeating, all of which may impair blood glucose regulation.

Maintaining a healthy glucose tolerance: requires a good night's sleep. Increased blood sugar levels result from impaired glucose tolerance, which is a condition in which the body struggles to digest and Organize your daily schedule and prioritize work to decrease

stress caused by time limits.

You can prevent feeling overwhelmed by breaking things into digestible components and setting reasonable goals.

Some useful tactics are as follows:

- Relaxation techniques: Engaging in relaxation techniques like yoga, progressive muscle relaxation, deep breathing exercises, or meditation can help lower stress and foster a sense of peace.

- Exercise and regular physical activity can help manage stress and improve blood glucose management, in addition to other health benefits. Your healthcare provider can help you choose the best workout program for you.

- Organize your daily schedule and prioritize work to decrease stress caused by time limits. You can prevent feeling overwhelmed by breaking things into digestible components and setting reasonable goals.

- Social support: Keep up a solid network of family, friends, or support organizations. Sharing your worries and emotions with people who can relate to your situation might

  help you feel better emotionally and reduce stress.

Discover and use the healthy coping methods that are most effective for you. This could be taking up hobbies, practicing mindfulness, keeping a journal, enjoying music, or engaging in other enjoyable and unwinding activities.

Take care of your emotional health by enlisting the aid of a professional, if necessary. Tools for controlling stress and enhancing general mental health can be found in therapy or counseling.

- Self-care: Give priority to self-care practices including getting enough sleep, eating balanced diet, and doing things that make you happy and relax you.

Keep in mind that it's crucial to speak with medical professionals, such as doctors, diabetes educators, or dietitians, who can offer specific guidance and help in managing stress and keeping stable blood glucose levels. They can assist with developing methods that are unique to your needs and assist in tracking your success.

Stress Management and Blood Glucose Harmony

Stress and blood sugar levels have a complicated link that varies from person to person. Particularly for those who have diabetes or are at risk for developing it, stress can affect blood sugar levels.

People can enhance their ability to control blood sugar levels and manage their diabetes more effectively by putting effective stress reduction techniques into practice, attending to their emotional needs, and building good coping mechanisms.

To manage stress and maintain stable blood sugar levels, keep in mind to seek the advice and assistance of healthcare professionals.

For people with diabetes in particular, stress management is essential for establishing stable blood sugar levels.

The production of chemicals like cortisol and adrenaline, which can raise blood sugar, is triggered by stress, and this can have a major effect on blood glucose levels.

Hormonal responses, increased appetite, and disturbance of routine are some ways that stress affects blood sugar levels.

Stress-related hormones like cortisol and adrenaline increase blood sugar levels by boosting hepatic glucose production and lowering insulin sensitivity. In addition to increasing the appetite for calorie- and carbohydrate-rich foods, stress can also cause overeating and high blood sugar levels. Stressful circumstances can also interfere with normal activities like eating, exercising, and taking medications, which can cause blood sugar levels to fluctuate. People may turn to emotional eating as a coping method during stressful times. Consuming comfort meals that are heavy in sugar and carbohydrates and cause blood sugar spikes is a common part of this practice. Additionally, people may engage in fewer self-care rituals, such as skipping workouts, getting enough sleep, and checking their blood sugar levels.

Blood sugar levels that are out of control may be influenced by these elements.

Blood sugar regulation and general health depend on managing stress

Here are some methods for reducing stress and preserving stable blood sugar levels:

1.Regular physical activity: Exercise and physical activity regularly can help lower stress and improve blood sugar regulation.

2.Relaxation methods: Using relaxation methods like yoga, deep breathing exercises, meditation, or mindfulness can help lower stress and foster a sense of peace.

3.choose healthy coping strategies: Find healthy coping strategies to deal with stress, such as journaling, talking to a supportive friend or family

member, partaking in hobbies, or, if necessary, getting professional assistance.

4.Eating a well-balanced diet that contains plenty of fruits, vegetables, whole grains, lean proteins, and healthy fats is important. Avoid consuming too many sugary or high-carbohydrate foods, particularly when under stress.

5.**Maintain a routine:** To help with improved blood sugar control and stress reduction, establish regular meal times, medication regimens, and sleep patterns.

6. **Put self-care first:** Look after yourself by getting enough sleep, participating in activities you enjoy, and making time for rest and self-care

Nurturing healthy weight management

Controlling one's weight is crucial for blood sugar regulation. People can increase their body's sensitivity to insulin and improve glucose control by maintaining a healthy weight. Insulin resistance is a disorder where the body's cells become less responsive to insulin, resulting in higher blood sugar levels. Excess weight, especially abdominal fat, is linked to this condition. It is possible to improve glucose utilization, lessen insulin resistance, and improve blood sugar control by losing weight with a combination of a balanced diet, consistent exercise, and lifestyle changes.

Additionally, weight-management techniques including portion control, picking foods high in

nutrients, and avoiding added sweets might help people achieve and maintain stable blood sugar levels. For those who have diabetes or are at risk of developing it, working is crucial. Management emphasizes maintaining a healthy body composition, which includes a desirable ratio of lean muscle mass to body fat, rather than just focusing on getting to a certain number on the scale. It is significant to remember that managing one's weight requires a long-term strategy rather than a -fix or fad diet. To promote progressive and stable weight loss or weight maintenance, if that is the goal sustainable lifestyle adjustments are encouraged.

Successful weight control also takes into account personal characteristics including age, sex, genetics, health issues, and lifestyle choices. It entails creating healthy routines, using portion control, tracking outcomes, and adjusting as appropriate to maintain weight or, if necessary, lose weight gradually.

Adopting a holistic strategy for sustaining a healthy weight and encouraging general well-being is necessary to foster healthy weight management.

It focuses on long-term lifestyle improvements that include balanced nutrition, consistent exercise, mindful eating, and emotional well-being.

The process of fostering healthy weight control takes time, patience, and consistency. The focus should be placed on implementing a balanced and long-term strategy that enhances overall health and well-being.

A diet that is well-balanced and rich in nutrients should emphasize a range of entire foods, such as fruits, vegetables, whole grains, lean meats, and healthy fats. This assists in supplying important nutrients while limiting calorie intake. Foods heavy in added sugars, saturated fats, and processed components should be avoided or limited.

This assists in supplying important nutrients while limiting calorie intake. Foods heavy in added sugars, saturated fats, and processed components should be avoided or limited.

Portion control: Be mindful of the sizes of food served to avoid overeating. To better manage portion control, be aware of serving sizes and employ strategies like utilizing smaller plates, monitoring meal portions, and mindful eating.
Hydration: Drink plenty of water throughout the day. Staying hydrated can help maintain overall health and support healthy weight management.

It can also help prevent confusion between thirst and hunger, as sometimes thirst is mistaken for food cravings. Recognizing symptoms and warning signs

Note: These symptoms can vary from person to person, and some individuals may not experience any noticeable symptoms.

Regular monitoring of blood sugar levels is crucial for accurate diagnosis and management of diabetes. If you experience persistent symptoms, it's ideal to consult a healthcare professional for proper evaluation and guidance

Monitoring and recognizing symptoms and warning signs of abnormal blood sugar levels is crucial for individuals with diabetes or those at risk of developing diabetes. Here are some common symptoms and warning signs associated with both high (hyperglycemia) and low (hypoglycemia) blood sugar levels

Ideas for breakfast that are suitable for diabetics

It's crucial to concentrate on meals that are low in carbohydrates, high in fiber, and contain lean protein when coming up with breakfast suggestions for diabetics.

Here are a few quick and wholesome breakfast suggestions:

1. Make a veggie omelet by using egg whites or a mixture of whole eggs and egg whites. Spinach, bell peppers, onions, and tomatoes are just a few examples of the colorful vegetables you can add. You can add some low-fat cheese for flavor as well.

2. Plain Greek yogurt with berries is a good choice because it is high in protein and low in carbs. Add a few strawberries, blueberries, or raspberries on top for decoration. To add more crunch and good fats, sprinkle some chopped nuts or seeds.

3. Avocado toast: Choose your favorite book or a low-carb substitute and spread mashed avocado on top.

 Add a squeeze of lemon juice, some salt, and pepper for flavor. For more protein, you could also sprinkle some tomatoes or a poached egg on top.

4. Smoothies: Blend unsweetened almond milk or Greek yogurt, a small amount of low-glycemic fruits like berries or half a banana, a scoop of protein powder,
and a handful of spinach or kale. Look for low-sugar varieties. This is a wholesome, quick, and simple breakfast alternative.

5. Chia seed pudding: Combine chia seeds with coconut milk or almond milk that hasn't been sweetened. Add a little amount of sugar-free sweetener or natural sweeteners like stevia or monk fruit extract. In the morning, sprinkle fresh berries or sliced almonds on top after the mixture has chilled overnight in the refrigerator.

6. Cottage cheese with tomatoes and cucumbers: Mix cottage cheese with thinly sliced tomatoes, cucumber, and a dash of basil or dill. It's a tasty, high-protein alternative for breakfast

How can I be tested for diabetes?

It's essential to speak with a healthcare provider if you have diabetes symptoms or wish to get tested as a preventative action. They'll be in a position to assess your symptoms, and risk factors, and arrange the necessary testing. I can, however, provide you with some general information on how diabetes is usually identified:

1. **Make an appointment:** Make an appointment with your primary care doctor or a medical professional with expertise in managing diabetes, like an endocrinologist.

2. **Medical History and Physical Exam:** Your healthcare professional will inquire about your medical history at your appointment, including any symptoms you may be feeling. They will also perform a physical examination to look for problems or indications of diabetes.

3. **Blood Measurement:** Measurements of blood glucose levels are one of the most frequent tests used to identify diabetes. Blood glucose tests come in a variety of forms:

You must fast for at least 8 hours before having your blood drawn for the fasting plasma glucose (FPG) test. In the morning, before you eat anything, it checks your blood sugar level.

How can I be tested for diabetes?

It's essential to speak with a healthcare provider if you have diabetes symptoms or wish to get tested as a preventative action. They'll be in a position to assess your symptoms, and risk factors, and arrange the necessary testing. I can, however, provide you with some general information on how diabetes is usually identified:

1. Make an appointment: Make an appointment with your primary care doctor or a medical professional with expertise in managing diabetes, like an endocrinologist.

2. Medical History and Physical Exam: Your healthcare professional will inquire about your medical history at your appointment, including any symptoms you may be feeling. They will also perform a physical examination to look for problems or indications of diabetes.

3. Blood Measurement: Measurements of blood glucose levels are one of the most frequent tests used to identify diabetes. Blood glucose tests come in a variety of forms:

You must fast for at least 8 hours before having your blood drawn for the fasting plasma glucose (FPG) test. In the morning, before you eat anything, it checks your blood sugar level.

Oral Glucose Tolerance Test (OGTT): For this test, you first fast before having your blood sugar levels checked, and then you consume a sweet beverage.
To determine how your body is metabolizing glucose, your blood sugar levels are reassessed after a few hours.

Regardless of when you last ate, the random plasma glucose test can be performed at any time. Your blood is measured.

4. Tests for glycated hemoglobin (A1C) and glucose levels: examine the average blood sugar levels over the previous two to three months.

It gives you a comprehensive view of your blood glucose control and does not require you to fast.

5. More testing: In a few instances, your doctor could advise more testing, such as a urine test to screen for ketones or autoantibodies linked to diabetes.

Diabetes-related health problems

Diabetes is a long-term medical illness that interferes with the body's ability to control blood sugar or glucose. If it is not adequately controlled, it can cause several health issues and consequences.

Diabetes can lead to several potential health issues, including:

1. Cardiovascular problems: Diabetes greatly raises the risk of cardiac problems, heart attacks, strokes, and high blood pressure. Blood vessels can be harmed by high blood sugar levels, which can also cause atherosclerosis, a condition in which the arteries constrict and stiffen.

2. Kidney disease:

Diabetic nephropathy, often known as diabetic nephropathy, is a primary cause of kidney disease. Over time, high blood sugar levels can harm the kidneys' small blood capillaries, reducing their capacity to remove waste and extra fluid from the body. Chronic renal disease may develop from this and call for dialysis or a kidney transplant.

3. Eye issues: Diabetic retinopathy, which affects the blood vessels in the retina, is one of many eye complications that can be brought on by the disease. If neglected, it may result in vision loss or blindness. A higher risk of glaucoma and cataracts is linked to diabetes.

4. **Nerve damage (neuropathy):** High blood sugar levels that persist over an extended period can harm the nerves throughout the body, resulting in a variety of neuropathies. Pain, tingling, numbness, and a lack of sensation are frequent symptoms of diabetic neuropathy in the feet and legs. Other organs may also be impacted, which may result in complications with the urinary system, the endocrine system, and the digestive system.

5. Complications relating to the feet: Diabetes can result in poor blood circulation and decreased sensation in the feet, leaving them more susceptible to infections, ulcers, and slowly healing wounds. If infections grow untreatable, severe cases may need to be amputated.

6. Skin issues: Diabetes can make skin more prone to infections, especially bacterial and fungal infections. Diabetes patients frequently experience dry skin, itching, and slowly healing wounds.

7. Dental problems: Gum conditions including gingivitis and periodontitis are made more likely by diabetes. Additionally, it may cause dry mouth, which increases the risk of cavities, foul breath, and oral infections.

What type of diabetes is riskier?

All forms of diabetes have some level of risk, but type 1 and type 2 diabetes are the most well-known and potentially dangerous forms.

Here is a quick rundown of their dangers:

1. **Type 1 diabetes:** This autoimmune disorder develops when the immune system unintentionally targets and kills the pancreatic cells that make insulin.

Insulin therapy is necessary for type 1 diabetics to survive.

Type 1 diabetes has several risks, including:

- Diabetic ketoacidosis (DKA): In the absence of insulin, the body begins to break down lipids for energy instead of appropriately processing glucose, which results in the creation of ketones. DKA, a condition that can be fatal, can be brought on by high ketones

- Hypoglycemia: Insulin therapy poses the danger of low blood sugar levels, which can lead to confusion, loss of consciousness, fainting, dizziness, and, in extreme cases, coma or death.

Poorly controlled type 1 diabetes can result in long-term issues including cardiovascular disease, renal damage, nerve damage, visual problems, and an elevated risk of infections.

2. Type 2 Diabetes: This disorder arises when the body develops insulin resistance or fails to produce enough insulin to keep blood sugar levels within normal range. It is frequently linked to lifestyle elements like obesity and inactivity, while genetics also play a part.

Type 2 diabetes has several risks, including:

- **Cardiovascular complications:** People with type 2 diabetes are at an increased risk of developing heart disease, stroke, and other cardiovascular issues.

- **Nerve damage:** Chronically elevated blood sugar levels can harm nerves, resulting in neuropathy, which can cause pain, numbness, and tingling in the extremities.

- **Kidney disease:** One of the main causes of kidney failure is diabetes.

- **Eye issues:** Diabetic retinopathy, cataracts, and glaucoma are more prevalent among diabetics.

Slow wound healing: Elevated blood sugar levels can interfere with the body's capacity to treat wounds, which can result in infections and other issues.

CHAPTER 6

Understanding signs and symptoms

It's significant to remember that these symptoms might differ from person to person, and some people may not experience any obvious symptoms. For an appropriate diabetes diagnosis and treatment plan, regular blood sugar monitoring is essential. It's crucial to speak with a medical practitioner for a proper assessment and recommendations if you have persistent or severe symptoms.

Symptoms of Blood Sugar levels

For people with diabetes or those who are at risk of getting the disease, monitoring and detecting symptoms and warning indications of elevated blood sugar levels are essential.

Here are some typical indications and symptoms of high (hyperglycemia) and low (hypoglycemia) blood sugar levels:

High Blood Sugar (Hyperglycemia) Symptoms

- **Frequent Urine:** Increased blood sugar levels can make the kidneys work harder, which results in more frequent urine.

Frequent urine can cause the body to become dehydrated, which can result in increased thirst.

- **Fatigue**: Having high blood sugar levels might make you feel exhausted and under-energized.

Dehydration brought on by elevated blood sugar levels might result in dry skin and itchy lips and tongue.

- **Vision haze:** Variations in blood sugar levels may have an impact on the eye's lens, resulting in momentary vision haze.

- **Wounds that take a long time to heal:** High blood sugar levels might make it harder for the body to get rid of infections and wounds.

Despite having high blood sugar levels, some people may still notice an increase in hunger.

- **Skin itchiness and dry mouth:** A dry mouth and itchy, dry skin might be symptoms of dehydration brought on by high blood sugar levels.

- **Increased appetite**: Despite not eating more, some people may nevertheless feel more hungry.

The complete approach to controlling your blood sugar

Schools, neighborhood associations, hospitals, and online platforms are just a few of the places where health education and awareness campaigns can be carried out. Health education and awareness help people feel better about themselves and their communities by generating knowledge, encouraging healthy behaviors, and empowering people.

You must collaborate with your healthcare provider to create a customized management plan because everyone has distinct demands.

Keep a close eye on your blood sugar levels, be proactive, and seek medical help as needed.

For people with diabetes or those who are at risk of getting the disease, controlling blood sugar levels is essential.

Here is a detailed plan to assist you in managing and controlling your blood sugar:

1. Eating Well: Consume a well-balanced diet that is high in whole grains, lean proteins, fruits, vegetables, and healthy fats.

2. Medication and Insulin: Follow your healthcare provider's instructions while taking any prescription drugs.

- If you need insulin, carefully adhere to the dosage and injection methods advised.

- Regularly check your blood sugar levels and modify the dosage of any medications or insulin as necessary.

3.Weight management: Keep your weight within a healthy range or strive to do so.

- If you are overweight, losing excess weight can greatly enhance blood sugar regulation.

4. Routine Checkup: Schedule routine medical checkups with your healthcare professional to monitor your blood sugar levels, evaluate your general health, and make any required modifications to your treatment plan.

5.Education and Support: Become knowledgeable about diabetes, how it is managed, and lifestyle changes.

- Participate in support groups or seek counseling to meet people dealing with comparable issues.
- Keep up with current techniques and breakthroughs in blood sugar management.

Guidelines

When the blood Sugar levels is out of range, a doctor will tell the patients what to do.

For a patient with diabetes, a doctor might suggest greater blood sugar objectives than for a patient without diabetes.

The day's target levels change. They typically peak an hour or so after meals and are typically lower just before and just after activity.

<u>**A doctor will take into account unique facts like the following when determining a patient's glucose targets**</u>:

- life expectancy and age
- the existence of additional medical problems, especially cardiovascular disease
- how long a person has had diabetes
- personal habits and lifestyle factors
- how conscious a person can be about diabetes.

<u>Special Considerations: Blood Glucose and Specific Condition</u>

Blood glucose levels need to be carefully monitored under certain circumstances.

Here are a few instances:

Diabetes: Elevated blood glucose levels are a defining feature of the disease. Type 1 and type 2 diabetics, in particular, must carefully control their blood sugar levels. This frequently entails regular blood glucose testing, adherence to a balanced diet, consistent exercise, and, occasionally, the use of insulin or prescription medication.

To create a customized management plan for people with diabetes, it's essential to collaborate closely with medical professionals.

High blood sugar levels are a defining feature of gestational diabetes, which develops throughout pregnancy. To protect the welfare of both the mother and the child, it necessitates constant monitoring and control. Gestational diabetic women may need to adhere to a special diet, check their blood sugar levels, exercise, and, in some situations, take medication or insulin. For optimal management, close communication with healthcare professionals is necessary.

Hypoglycemia: Low blood sugar levels are referred to as hypoglycemia. People with diabetes who take insulin or specific diabetes medicines may experience it. It can also occur in persons without diabetes as a result of other underlying medical issues or binge drinking. Consuming fast-acting carbs, such as those found in fruit juice or glucose pills, can help manage hypoglycemia by swiftly raising blood sugar levels. It's critical to recognize the signs of hypoglycemia and act appropriately to avoid complications.

Hyperglycemia: is a term for high blood sugar levels that is frequently used to describe diabetics whose blood glucose levels are persistently higher. Long-term problems might result from uncontrolled hyperglycemia. Following a specified diabetes management plan is necessary to control hyperglycemia. This strategy may include altering insulin dosages or medication, routinely checking blood glucose levels, and changing one's lifestyle to include a nutritious diet and frequent exercise.

Polycystic Ovary Syndrome: FC Blood glucose level can be impacted by several medical illnesses, including polycystic ovarian syndrome (PCOS), metabolic syndrome, and certain hormonal abnormalities. To address their blood sugar control and general health, people with certain diseases may need particular treatment measures. It's crucial to collaborate with medical experts who can offer advice.

Managing Diabetes in Children and Adolescents

The diabetes treatment strategy for each child should be customized to meet their unique requirements, preferences, and developmental stage. Successful diabetes management in children and adolescents can be facilitated by regular communication and cooperation between the kid, their family, medical providers, and the school.

Diabetes education is crucial to raise awareness of the disease among children and their caregivers. Knowing how to check blood sugar, administer insulin (if necessary), plan meals, and identify high- or low-blood-sugar symptoms are all included in this. Healthcare experts, such as diabetes educators or pediatric endocrinologists, can give diabetes education.

- **Blood Sugar Monitoring:** It's essential to regularly check your blood sugar levels if you want to manage diabetes in kids and teenagers. Using a glucose meter or continuous glucose monitoring (CGM) devices, blood sugar levels must be checked several times each day to achieve this. The outcomes support modifying insulin dosages and selecting the best food and exercise options

- **Insulin Management**: For children and adolescents with type 1 diabetes or in certain situations, type 2 diabetes, insulin treatment may be required. The healthcare team for child will choose the best insulin regimen, which may entail insulin pump therapy or numerous daily injections. Training on insulin delivery methods and dosage modification should be provided for parents and carers.

To manage diabetes in kids, you should keep certain things in mind

- **Food preparation:** It's critical to create a balanced, personal food plan for each kid or adolescent with diabetes. To develop a meal plan that satisfies nutritional requirements, controls blood sugar levels, and takes into account the child's preferences and lifestyle, work with a registered dietitian with experience in pediatric diabetes. To maintain constant blood sugar control, it's crucial to set regular meal and snack periods.

- **Support on an emotional level:** Children and teenagers who have diabetes may find it difficult to do so. Assist them emotionally and foster an environment where they feel free to express their worries or annoyances. As kids become increasingly capable of taking care of themselves, promote open communication and include them in the decisions about how to manage their diabetes.

- **Support from the school:** Work together to develop a diabetes control strategy with the kid's school. This may entail educating school personnel on managing diabetes, assuring access to blood sugar monitoring and insulin delivery, making accommodations for meals and snacks, and supporting the kid during physical activities.

- **Regular Medical Checkups:** Arrange regular follow-up appointments with the child's healthcare team to track the management of the child's diabetes, evaluate general health, modify treatment plans as necessary, and address any problems.

- **Encourage frequent exercise as part of your diabetes control strategy.**

Exercise assists in weight management, improves general health, and helps control blood sugar levels Work together with the medical staff to identify the appropriate levels of activity, and change insulin dosages or food intake as needed to maintain blood sugar stability during exercise.

Diabetes injury hazards

A diabetic who has an accident must consider several variables, including the injury's seriousness, the person's general health, and how effectively their diabetes is controlled.

However, there are a few prevalent things to recognize:

1. **Delayed Healing:** Because diabetes impairs blood circulation and compromises immunological function, it might impede the body's capacity to repair wounds. High blood sugar levels can delay healing, making it more difficult to complete.

2. **Enhanced Risk of Infection:** Diabetes can impair immune function, leaving sufferers more vulnerable to infections. A skin injury that breaks increases the likelihood of acquiring infections like cellulitis or even more catastrophic illnesses like sepsis.

3. **Poor blood sugar control:** Stress to the body from an injury or trauma can cause blood sugar levels to fluctuate. Blood sugar levels may rise as a result of stress hormone release, which makes maintaining ideal glucose control harder. On the other hand, if a person's appetite is hampered, they might not eat enough, which could result in low blood sugar levels.

4. **Nerve Damage:** Diabetes can result in neuropathy or damaged nerves. It may be more difficult to detect wounds or injuries in injured diabetics due to decreased sensation in the affected

area. As a result, individuals could delay getting immediate medical help, which can cause more problems.

5. **Consequences:** Serious consequences like ulcers, abscesses, or even cancer can develop if an injury gets infected or does not heal properly. In extreme circumstances, amputation can be required.

Food that can help in the healing process of a diabetic patient.

It is advised to keep a well-balanced diet because it will aid in overall health and the healing process, as there is no specific list of foods that will treat a diabetic injury.

Diets that can help people with diabetes are listed below.

1. Whole grains: Choose whole grains such as brown rice, quinoa, whole wheat bread, and whole grain cereals. These give you fiber and important nutrients that advance your general wellness.

2. Lean proteins: Include lean protein sources such as skinless fish, poultry, tofu, lentils, and legumes. Consuming enough protein helps the establishment of new blood vessels and tissue, which speeds up the recovery of diabetic wounds. Foods that are heavy in protein tend to be more filling than those that are high in carbohydrates or fat.

3. Fruits and vegetables: Incorporate a variety of colorful fruits and vegetables into your diet. They are rich in antioxidants, vitamins, and minerals that support the immune system and overall healing.

4. Foods rich in vitamin C: Vitamin C is important for collagen production, which is essential for wound healing. Include citrus fruits, strawberries, kiwis, bell peppers, and broccoli in your diet. Vitamin C has been shown to enhance collateral vessel formation, improving blood supply to injured tissues. This effect can be particularly beneficial for diabetic patients with impaired wound healing or ischemic injuries.

5. Omega-3 fatty acids: Foods rich in omega-3 fatty acids, such as fatty fish (salmon, mackerel, and sardines), walnuts, flaxseeds, and chia seeds, have anti-inflammatory properties that can aid in the healing process.

6. Hydration:

Keep yourself well-hydrated at all times. Water is necessary for all cell functions, including those of the tissues that are healing. A healthy physique can help you manage your blood sugar levels more effectively. For those with diabetes, it's especially crucial to quench thirst and avoid dehydration through water consumption. To filter waste products, including glucose, the kidneys must work at their best, which can be maintained with adequate hydration.

Targeted blood Sugar Levels

Targeted blood sugar levels are the range of blood glucose concentrations that people with diabetes work to reach and maintain using a variety of management techniques, including medication, dietary changes, physical activity, and lifestyle adjustments.

These target values have been established to encourage ideal glycemic management and lower the possibility of issues brought on by either high or low blood sugar. The precise target blood sugar levels can change depending on a person's age, general health, the presence of multiple conditions, and treatment strategies.

Following are some typical target blood sugar levels for diabetics:

1. Fasting Blood Sugar:

- **Target Range:** For the majority of people with diabetes, the American Diabetes Association (ADA) advises a target fasting blood sugar level of 80–130 mg/dL (4.4–7.2 mmol/L) before meals.

- **Goal**: Maintaining a consistent fasting blood sugar level lowers the risk of hypo- or hyperglycemia and contributes to stable glucose control throughout the day.

2. Postprandial Blood Sugar (After Meal):

- **Target Range**: For the majority of people with diabetes, the ADA advises a target postprandial blood sugar level below 180 mg/dL (10.0 mmol/L), tested 1-2 hours after beginning a meal.
- **Goal**: Preventing excessive postprandial glucose spikes, which can lead to long-term problems and unstable glucose control, is made possible by controlling postprandial blood sugar levels.

3. Glycated hemoglobin HbA1c

- **Target Range:** For the majority of people with diabetes, the ADA generally advises a anbA1c target of less than 7%. However, based on variables including age, general health, and the risk of hypoglycemia, specific goals may be defined.

- **Goal**: The HbA1c test measures the average blood sugar levels over two to three months. Targeting a particular HbA1c level lowers the

  risk of problems brought on by persistently high blood sugar levels and aids in evaluating long-term glycemic management.

Target blood sugar levels may change depending on a person's circumstances, and medical practitioners may change particular targets to suit a person's requirements and medical background. To attain and maintain the goal blood sugar levels for optimal diabetes management, regular blood sugar monitoring and continual communication with healthcare experts are crucial. These actions allow you to assess your progress and make the required corrections.

CHAPTER 7

Long-Term Strategies for Maintaining Blood Sugar Control

For those with diabetes, controlling blood sugar levels is essential to avoiding problems and maintaining general health. Long-term blood sugar control success necessitates a multifaceted strategy that includes lifestyle modifications, medication management, and routine monitoring. In this booklet, I will examine an extensive guide to long-term methods for sustaining blood sugar control.

Lifestyle modification

The Importance of a Healthy Lifestyle:

The first step in effective blood sugar control is making lifestyle changes that support stable glucose levels. These modifications not only improve blood sugar control but also general health.

1. **Develop Healthy Eating Habits:** Emphasize a balanced diet that is full of whole grains, lean proteins, healthy fats, and a variety of fruits and vegetables.
To avoid overeating, which can cause blood sugar to surge, pay attention to portion sizes.
There should be a moderation in the consumption of processed foods, sugary beverages

2. **Regular Physical Activity:** Exercise regularly by jogging, cycling, swimming, or even just fast

walking to increase insulin sensitivity and lower blood sugar levels.

Aim for at least 150 minutes per week of moderate-intensity aerobic exercise and two times per week of muscle-strengthening activities.

3. **Weight Control:**

Reach a healthy weight and keep it there to improve insulin sensitivity and better control blood sugar.

Speak with a medical expert to create a customized plan and establish reasonable weight loss targets.

4. **Stress reduction:**

Use stress-reduction methods like yoga, meditation, deep breathing, and mindfulness to help reduce blood sugar increases brought on by stress.

medication and monitoring

Medication and monitoring: For simple check-ups and health management, it is advised that you engage with a healthcare expert. They are qualified to provide medications for your medical conditions.

1. Adherence to Medication: To ensure consistent blood sugar control, take prescription medications as instructed by your doctor. Tell your doctor about any worries or side effects so they can, if required, modify your treatment plan.

2. Insulin Administration: If insulin therapy is recommended, become knowledgeable about how to give it and how to handle dosage changes depending on blood sugar monitoring. Use an insulin pump as directed or stick to a regular schedule for insulin injections.

3. Drugs taken by mouth: If your treatment plan calls for oral drugs, take them as prescribed and check on their efficacy periodically with your doctor.

<u>Ongoing Education and Support</u>

Continuous Learning And Support Networks

1. Education on Diabetes

Enroll in diabetes education classes to gain a deeper understanding of the disease, control blood sugar, and adopt a healthy lifestyle.

Keep up with new developments in diabetes treatment by consulting reliable sources and professional literature.

2. Regular Examinations

Make regular consultations with your medical team to review your blood sugar management, make any required corrections, and discuss any issues.

3. Support Systems

Participate in online communities or diabetes support groups to meet people going through similar experiences.

To deal with the psychological effects of controlling diabetes, ask friends, family, and mental health specialists for emotional support.

4. Goal Setting - Establish attainable short- and long-term goals for controlling blood sugar, engaging in physical activity, and developing healthy eating habits. Maintaining attainable and motivating goals requires regular assessment and adjustment.

You can greatly enhance your long-term health results and have a satisfying life while successfully managing diabetes by incorporating these techniques into your everyday practice.

Monitoring And Adjusting Your Plans

A key component of treating and preventing diabetes is maintaining healthy blood sugar levels. Achieving and maintaining stable blood sugar levels, avoiding problems, and improving general wellbeing all depend heavily on monitoring and modifying your strategy.

Strategies for Adjusting Your Plan:

1. Recognizing Patterns: Examine your blood sugar records to find trends and patterns. Keep track of the effects that various foods, activities, stresses, and medications have on your levels. Post-meal rises, morning highs (the dawn phenomenon), and overnight dips (hypoglycemia) are typical trends.

2. Modifying Diet and Carbohydrate Intake: Diet is crucial for controlling blood sugar levels. Consider modifying your carbohydrate consumption based on the data from your monitoring. You may need to decrease your carbohydrate portion sizes or seek foods with a lower glycemic index if your post-meal readings are consistently high. On the other hand, if you have hypoglycemia, eating a modest snack might be beneficial.

3. Changing Physical Activity: Exercise helps control blood sugar levels when done regularly. Examine the effects of various workout regimens, lengths of time, and levels of intensity on your readings. Find a balance in your routine to avoid sharp drops or surges. Consider modifying your pre-exercise snack or insulin dosage if you experience hypoglycemia during or after exercise.

4. Medication and Insulin Adjustments: Monitoring is essential for people taking diabetic medication or receiving insulin therapy to ensure an adequate dose. Based on your blood sugar trends, your healthcare professional will advise you on how to change the dosage of your medications. Never change your

medicine without consulting a doctor, because doing so can cause problems.

5. Stress management: Prolonged stress can raise blood sugar levels by causing the production of cortisol and other chemicals. Consider adopting stress reduction strategies like mindfulness, meditation, or relaxation techniques to lessen the influence of stressors on your readings.

6. Blood sugar levels can be impacted by sleep hygiene and timing as well as by the quantity and quality of sleep: Keep track of how your readings change depending on your sleep patterns. Your levels might be positively impacted by regular sleep schedules and appropriate sleep hygiene habits.

Long-term sustainability and lifestyle modifications

Focus on implementing sustainable lifestyle changes while you monitor and optimize your plan. Gradual changes have a higher chance of sticking, and consistency is essential for long-lasting effects. Make an effort to establish a balanced schedule that includes adherence to your medicine, stress management, food, and exercise.

CONCLUSION

Keeping blood sugar levels steady is vital for overall health and well-being. Elevated or low blood sugar levels can lead to various complications and health risks, particularly for individuals with diabetes. Individuals can effectively regulate their blood sugar levels by adopting a balanced and healthy lifestyle which includes regular exercise, nutritious food, adequate medication (if necessary), and regular monitoring. Instead of consuming most of your protein in a single meal, distribute your protein intake evenly throughout the day. Planning your meals and snacks can help you achieve a balanced macronutrient intake. Aim to include a source of protein, carbohydrates, and fats in each meal and snack to ensure a well-rounded nutritional profile.This approach helps optimize muscle protein synthesis and provides a steady supply of amino acids to support various bodily functions.

It is also critical to seek specific guidance and support from healthcare specialists. Taking proactive steps to maintain appropriate blood sugar levels supports good physical and mental functioning and lowers the risk of long-term consequences linked with blood sugar abnormalities. Remember that tiny modifications in everyday behaviors can make a big impact in obtaining and maintaining **stable blood**

sugar levels, which can help you lose weight. Discover and use the healthy coping methods that are most effective for you. This could be taking up hobbies, practicing mindfulness, keeping a journal, enjoying music, or engaging in other enjoyable and unwinding activities. Also, Make it a habit to study product labels to detect hidden sugars in packaged goods. High fructose corn syrup, sucrose, dextrose, and other kinds of added sugars should be avoided. Choose sugar-free foods or natural sweeteners such as stevia or monk fruit. Aim for meals that are well-balanced and contain a variety of carbs, proteins, and healthy fats. Combining protein and fat with carbohydrates can aid in reducing the pace of sugar digestion and absorption, resulting in more stable blood sugar levels. Include healthy fats from foods like avocados, nuts, seeds, and olive oil as well as lean proteins from sources like poultry, fish, tofu, and lentils. Drink enough water throughout the day to stay well hydrated. Avoid sugary beverages and too much caffeine because they can impact your blood sugar levels and level of hydration. The transportation of glucose and glycogen into our body's tissues for utilization as fuel is dependent on our bloodstream. When glucose reaches the appropriate tissues through our blood and the circulatory system, it starts to disintegrate. Because of this, the amount of glucose that is present in the blood is referred to as blood glucose.

Remember that every person's nutritional requirements are unique, so it's vital to speak with a registered dietitian or another healthcare provider who can offer tailored advice based on your unique health objectives and medical conditions. They can facilitate the development of a balanced food plan that fits your lifestyle and promotes the best blood sugar regulation.